# EASY TO

# *RENAL DIET*

## COOKBOOK

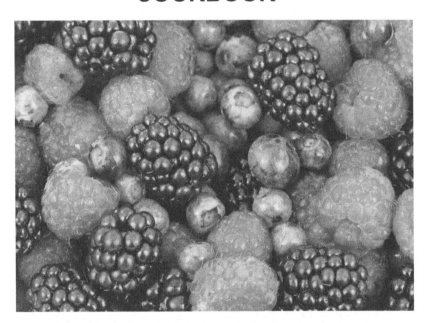

## ONLY LOW SODIUM, LOW POTASSIUM, LOW PHOSPHORUS HEALTHY RECIPES TO AVOID DIALYSIS!

# TABLE OF CONTENTS

# *Introduction*

Kidney (or renal) diseases are affecting around 14% of the adult population according to international stats. In the US, approx. 661.000 Americans suffer from kidney dysfunction. Out of these patients, 468.000 proceed to dialysis treatment and the rest have one active kidney transplant.

The high numbers of diabetes and heart disease are also correlated with kidney dysfunction and sometimes one condition e.g. diabetes may lead to the other.

With so many high rates, perhaps the best course of treatment is the prevention of dialysis, which makes people depend on clinical and hospital treatments at least two times a week. Therefore, if your kidney has already shown some signs of dysfunction, you can prevent dialysis through diet, something that we are going to discuss in this book.

# *What is Kidney Disease?*

A kidney disease diagnosis implies that the kidneys are either dysfunctioning, under-functioning or damaged and cannot filter out toxins and metabolic waste on their own. Our systems need our kidneys for a waste filtering process. However, when kidney damage occurs, the system is piled up with damaging waste that it cannot expel through other means. As a result, inflammatory responses emerge and you have a much higher chance of developing chronic and serious health disorders like diabetes or heart failure, which can even be fatal in extreme cases.

There are two main types of kidney disease, based on their cause and time duration:

- **Sudden and unexpected kidney damage/acute kidney injury (AKI)** as a result of an accident or surgery side effects, which usually lasts for a short period of time.

- **Chronic and progressive kidney dysfunction (CKD).** As its name suggests, this is a chronic condition with multiple progressive stages that lead ultimately to permanent kidney damage. There are approx. 5 stages of the disorder and during the last and final stage, the patient will need dialysis or a kidney transplant to survive. This final stage is also known in the medical glossary as End-Stage-Renal Disease (ESRD).

During all kidney dysfunction stages, there are higher than normal amounts of a certain protein called *Arbutin* in the urine, which can be confirmed by urine tests for diagnosing renal disease. This condition is known scientifically as *Proteinuria*. Doctors may also perform blood tests and/or image screening tests to pinpoint a problem with the kidneys and come up with a diagnosis.

# What are the causes of Kidney Disease?

Chronic kidney disease is often the result of other chronic health conditions. Diabetes, according to medical stats, is the leading cause of kidney dysfunction and ultimately ESRD. Other common causes include:

- Elevated blood pressure
- Autoimmune problems and disorders such as Lupus, celiac disease and IgA neuropathy.
- Urinary tract problems and infections
- Nephrotic syndrome (a condition that results in abnormal levels of protein in the urine while the actual protein levels in the blood are low).

In some cases, kidneys may cease to function unexpectedly for a very brief period of time that is usually a couple of days. This is the result of an accident or sudden body failures like:

- Heart Attack
- Drug and substance abuse
- Insufficient blood flow to the kidneys
- Urinary tract infections

In this case, the kidney damage is only temporary and your kidneys will switch back to their normal function after just a couple days, especially if you don't have any other chronic health problems that will affect their recovery.

The problem is, kidney damage at first doesn't show any symptoms that you can notice on your own and it's no wonder why many people call it a "silent disease". The symptoms usually are more noticeable during the last stages of the disease and include:

- Fatigue for no reason
- Feeling of coldness and numbness
- Breath problems e.g. shortness of breath
- Weakness and tiredness
- Dizziness, nausea

- Cognitive problems e.g. trouble concentrating and thinking clearly
- Swelling of hands and feet
- Swelling and puffiness or redness in the face
- Change in taste sensations/food appears to have a metal taste.
- Ammonia/bad breath
- Tendency to vomit
- Itchiness
- Bubbly and burning urine
- Red, brown or purple urine
- Intense pressure needed to urinate

Many of the above symptoms though can be a sign of other health conditions e.g. inflammatory bowel disease and so if you have any of the above mentioned, you have to consult with a doctor for a proper diagnosis and before the condition gets worse.

# Renal Diet and its Benefits

If you have been diagnosed with kidney dysfunction, a proper diet is necessary for controlling the amount of toxic waste in the bloodstream. When toxic waste piles up in the system along with increased fluid, chronic inflammation occurs and we have a much higher chance of developing cardiovascular, bone, metabolic or other health issues.

Since your kidneys can't fully get rid of waste on their own, which comes from food and drinks, probably the only natural way to help our system is through this diet.

A renal diet is especially useful during the first stages of kidney dysfunction and leads to the following benefits:

- Prevents excess fluid and waste build-up
- Prevents the progression of renal dysfunction stages

- Decreases the likelihood of developing other chronic health problems e.g. heart disorders
- Has a mild antioxidant function in the body, which keeps inflammation and inflammatory responses under control.

The above-mentioned benefits are noticeable once the patient follows the diet for at least a month and then continuing it for longer periods, to avoid the stage where dialysis is needed. The strictness of the diet depends on the current stage of renal/kidney disease, if, for example, you are in the 3rd or 4th stage, you should follow a more strict diet and be attentive for the food, which is allowed or prohibited.

These exact foods and nutrients that you should take when following a renal diet, will be given to you in the following sections, so keep on reading.

## Explanation of key diet words

The following nutrients play a major role in the renal diet as some have the ability to improve the condition while others can make it worse. Essentially, renal diet is based on low consumption of certain nutrients like potassium and phosphorus simply because it promotes fluid buildup within the system of a kidney patient. Here is a brief explanation of the function of each nutrient and its role in a renal diet:

## Potassium.

Potassium is a mineral that naturally occurs in certain foods and plays a role in regulating heart rhythm and muscle movement. It is also needed for keeping fluid and electrolyte balance in normal levels. Our kidneys keep only the right levels of potassium in our system, and when it is excess, they expel it via the urine.

The problem is, once kidneys can't function properly, all this excess potassium can't be expelled out and spikes up, causing symptoms like muscle and bone weakness, abnormal heartbeat, and heart failure in extreme cases. Thus, a diet low in potassium is recommended to prevent buildup and avoid such negative side effects.

**Sodium.**

Sodium is a trace mineral that is found in most foods that we eat today and it is the key component of salt, which is actually a sodium compound mixed with chloride. Most food that we consume and especially processed food is highly loaded with salt, however, we may be eating sodium in other forms too e.g. fish. The key role of sodium is to regulate blood pressure, help regulate nerve function, and maintain the balance of acids in the blood. However, when sodium is excessively high and the kidneys can expel it, it can lead to the following symptoms: an elevated feeling of thirst, swelling of hands, feet and the face, elevated blood pressure, and problems with breathing.

This is why it is suggested to keep sodium intake low, to avoid the above.

**Phosphorus.**

Phosphorus is an essential mineral that is responsible for the development and regeneration of our bones. Phosphorus also plays a key role in the growth of connective tissue e.g. muscles and the regulation of muscle motions. When food we take contains phosphorus, it gets absorbed by the intestines and then gets deposited in our bones.

However, when kidneys are damaged or dysfunctioning, the excess phosphorus can't be expelled through our systems and causes problems such as: extracting calcium out of the bones/making them weaker, and leading to excess calcium in the bloodstream which interferes with blood vessels, heart, eye, and lung function.

**Protein.**

Protein is a nutritional compound that consists of amino acids, which play a key role in various system functions like cell communication, oxygen supply, and cellular metabolism. They are also a part of a healthy immune system.

Normally, protein is not an issue for our kidneys. When protein is metabolized, waste by-products are also created and are filtered through the kidneys. This waste along with extra renal proteins after will be expelled through urine.

However, when kidneys are unable to filter out excess protein, it gets accumulated in the blood and cause problems.

This doesn't mean that renal disease patients should avoid protein totally as it is still necessary for some metabolic functions, as long as it's taken in moderate amounts and based on the stage of renal disease.

**Carbs.**

Carbs act as a key source of fuel for our bodies. The consumption of carbs is turned into glucose in our system, which is a primary source of energy.

Carbs are ok to be eaten in moderation by kidney patients and the daily recommended allowance is up to 150 grams/day. However, patients that also suffer from Diabetes (besides renal disease) should control their carb consumption to avoid any sudden spikes in their blood glucose.

**Fats.**

Being in balanced amounts, fats in our bodies act as an energy source, aid in the release of hormones, and help regulate blood pressure. They also carry some vitamins that are fat-soluble such as A, D, E, and K, which are also very important for our systems. Not all fats are created equal though, some are good for our health and some are bad. Bad fats are saturated and trans fats and are found in processed meat, dairy, and other products. They are also found in margarine and vegetable fat shortenings.

Fats, in general, don't pose a risk for renal disease patients, however, it is suggested to limit the consumption of saturated and trans fats to avoid any cardiovascular problems e.g. elevated blood pressure and clogging of the arteries.

**Dietary fiber.**

Dietary fiber is a compound that can't be digested on its own by enzymes and acids in our stomach and intestines but is needed for the system to aid in the digestion of our food and encourage bowel movements. They generally promote bowel regularity and decrease the likelihood of developing constipation inside the colon. Dietary fiber is typically found in fruits, vegetables, seeds, and whole grains.

In patients with renal disease, dietary fiber is ok up to 28 grams/day as long as these plant foods don't contain high amounts of phosphorus or potassium.

**Vitamins.**

According to medical and dietary guidelines, our bodies need close to 13 vitamins to functions. Vitamins play a key role in metabolic functions and the normal functioning of our cardiovascular, digestive, nervous system and immune systems. The adoption of a nutritionally dense and balanced diet is necessary for getting all the vitamins our system needs. However, due to some diet restrictions e.g. sodium, many renal patients are in need of water-soluble vitamins like B-complex (B1, B2, B6, B12, folic acid, biotin) and small amounts of Vitamin C.

**Minerals.**

Minerals are needed for our system to maintain healthy connective tissue e.g. bones, muscles, and skin and facilitate the normal function of our hearts and central nervous systems.

Our kidneys typically expel any excess amount of minerals through our urine as some can lead to health symptoms e.g. muscle spasms when their levels are abnormally high.

However, as it was mentioned earlier, some minerals like potassium and phosphorus cannot be expelled by our kidneys when in excess and so their intake through diet should be limited.

Other trace minerals are perfectly fine when following a renal diet: iron, copper, zinc, and selenium. A lack of these can lead to increased oxidative stress and thus, it is important to take sufficient amounts through diet or supplementation.

**Fluids.**

Fluids are necessary for the proper hydration of our systems in fact; lack of fluids can lead to dehydration and death in extreme cases.

However, in patients with renal dysfunction, fluids can quickly build up to the point of placing pressure to vital organs like the lungs and heart and becoming dangerous. This is the reason why many physicians advise their kidney patients to limit the consumption of fluids, especially during the last stages of the disorder.

# *What to Eat and What to Avoid in Renal Diet*

As specified above, some nutrients should be limited in renal diet e.g. phosphorus, potassium, and thus any foods that contain high amounts of these should be taken only in low amounts and not on a daily basis. The foods that should be limited are:

- Bananas
- Avocadoes
- Beetroots
- Dried beans
- Dried fruit
- Mangos
- Melons
- Molasses
- Nuts and seeds
- Oranges
- Parsnips
- Spinach
- Potatoes
- Fish
- Low-fat yogurt

Be attentive! Following foods have a high amount of sodium and their consumption should be limited:

- Salty snacks e.g. pretzels, potato chips, packed popcorn etc.

- Savory pies e.g. cheese pies, sausage rolls, and Greek spinach pies
- Processed meats e.g. luncheon meat, salami, sausages
- Pickled foods in salt brine
- Condiments e.g. ketchup, mustard, and mayo
- Soy sauce
- Canned soups and sauces

Now, here are the top foods you can consume without any (strict) restrictions, as they are naturally low in potassium, phosphorus, and sodium:

- Cabbage
- Cucumber
- Broccoli
- Cauliflower
- Brussels sprouts
- Onions
- Garlic
- Apples

- Berries (blueberries, cranberries, berries, strawberries)
- Cherries
- Red grapes
- Egg whites
- Wild caught fish
- Olive oil
- Bulgur wheat
- Oatmeal
- Skinless chicken and turkey
- Arugula
- Macadamia Nuts
- Radishes
- Shiitake mushrooms
- Pineapple
- Grapefruits
- Kale
- Ginger
- All spices and herbs

Red meat and dairy can also be consumed in moderation but they should not be combined with high phosphorus, potassium, or sodium foods as they contain moderate amounts of these alone.

# *List of Juices and Drinks for Renal Diet*

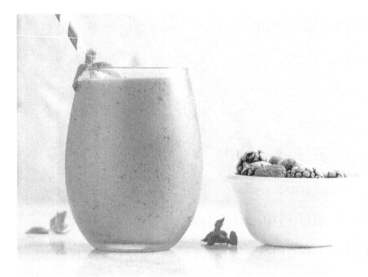

If you wish sufficiently hydrate yourself without increasing your sodium, phosphorus or potassium intake, there are a few drinks and juices you can drink on a regular basis:

- Freshly made apple juice
- Berry juices

- Red wine (up to two glasses a day)
- Grape juice
- Filtered drinking water
- Pineapple juice
- Cucumber juice
- Lemon juice diluted
- Most unsweetened herbal tea e.g. green tea, mint, ginger, cinnamon, etc.
- Coffee (in moderation)

During the late stages of renal dysfunction and particularly from stage 3, as usual, physicians recommend the limitation of fluids up to 1500 mg/day (which is equal to 5-6 glasses of liquids per day). However, this is something that you'd better discuss with your doctor as adjusting the amount yourself may lead to fluid imbalance.

# *Answers to Frequently Asked Questions*

When you diagnosed with renal disease, it is perfectly natural and common to have some questions in regards to kidney function and renal diet. Here are the most common questions and their answers in brief:

**Q: How much protein should I take daily?**

**A:** The exact amount of protein you should take per day depends on your existing body weight, stage of renal disease, and general health status. This is something that you can figure out with your doctor or renal dietitian. However, in most cases, doctors recommend the approx. 1.1-1.3 gr of protein per kg of body weight daily. For example, if you weight 143Pounds/65Kg, you can eat up to 84 grams of protein per day without any problems.

**Q: Do I need to take extra vitamins and supplements?**

**A:** Due to the fact that a lot of nutrient-dense foods should be avoided in the renal diet because of their high potassium or phosphorus content, it is generally suggested to take vitamins that are water soluble and namely B-complex vitamins and vitamin C in smaller doses. However, excess supplementation may lead to side effects like stomach irritation, gas and constipation so make sure you do not exceed the daily-recommended dose on the package.

**Q: Are alcoholic beverages ok to drink in a renal diet?**

**A:** Drinks that contain lower amounts of alcohol than others e.g. wine and beer are fine to drink on a semi-regular basis e.g. 2-3 times a week. However, heavy alcoholic drinks like vodka, rum, tequila, gin, and whiskey should be limited to 2-3 times a month, as frequent consumption will place kidneys and other vital organs under stress.

**Q: How can I figure out if a packed food product or recipe is low in potassium?**

**A:** When you are checking a product label or new recipe but don't know if it's actually low in potassium or not, here is a basic guideline of levels per serving:

| Very low potassium levels | up to 35 mg/serving |
|---|---|
| Low potassium levels | up to 150 mg/serving |
| Moderate potassium levels | Between 150-250 mg/serving |
| High potassium levels | 250-500 mg/serving |
| Very high potassium levels | 500mg+/serving |

If you are checking a recipe, make sure that you calculate the total levels of all ingredients to determine the amount of potassium. In this book, we made it easier for you by including recipes that are low or moderate in potassium and display the actual potassium level per serving.

**Q: Do I have to limit my fluids after being diagnosed?**

**A:** A limitation of fluids is generally recommended during the last stages of kidney damage and it would be better to discuss with your doctor. If you go opposite and only drink 500ml of fluids or less per day, you risk dehydrating yourself and cause other problems.

**Q: Are artificial sweeteners OK in renal diet?**

**A:** Artificial sweeteners that are low in carbs are generally fine to the consumer within the renal diet with the exception of aspartame which is linked to many health problems, sweeteners like stevia, sucralose, and xylitol are perfectly fine when consumed moderately on a regular basis.

**Q: Can I follow this diet if I have a kidney transplant?**

A: Although this diet is designed to help patients of nearly all stages of kidney damage, once you have a kidney transplant surgery, you may follow afterward a similar diet but your protein requirements will be higher, as your body will need extra protein to heal damaged tissue. In addition, maybe you will need to eat higher amounts of calcium to avoid any depletion because of steroid medications. The exact diet and portions are something that you will discuss with your doctor or renal dietician post-surgery.

# *Best Advice to Avoid Dialysis*

As specified, if you are currently in the first stages of renal damage, you can actually prevent dialysis mainly through diet, but there are other general lifestyle factors that will help. As a rule of thumb, you need to follow a lifestyle that keeps your body weight under control and makes you feel healthy. Here are some tips:

**Exercise on a regular basis.** It is important to be physically active to keep your heart and breathing system healthy, as renal damage can also affect their functions as well. Most doctors recommend exercising 2-3 times a week and performing mild exercises to keep yourself active but not too tired or exhausted. Three hours in total of mild exercise per week is perfectly fine for this purpose.

**Monitor your blood sugar levels.** Blood sugar levels and diabetes are often a side effect or even a contributing factor to renal damage. Even if you don't have currently diabetes, it is still important to monitor your blood sugar levels as they can place you at risk of developing renal disease further. Check them at least once a month and if you are in pre-diabetes or full set diabetes status, make sure that you take all the medicines that your doctor prescribes for your case.

**Keep your immune system balanced.** When our immune systems are underactive or overactive, many types of diseases can occur as a result of the body's inability to fight them in a proper manner. In the case of renal disease, some autoimmune conditions like Lupus are negatively associated with the progression of the disease. In this case, your doctor may prescribe steroids to keep your immune system from getting over-triggered and attacking vital organs e.g. kidneys.

# Recipes

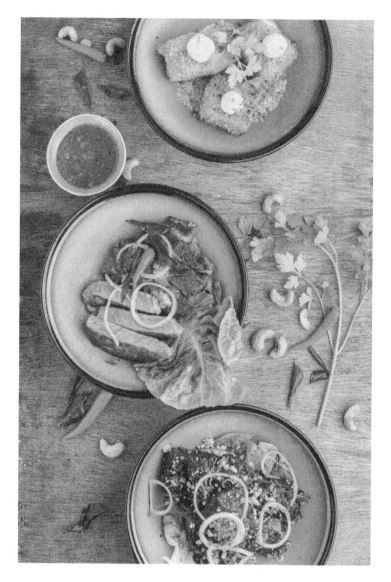

# *Breakfast*

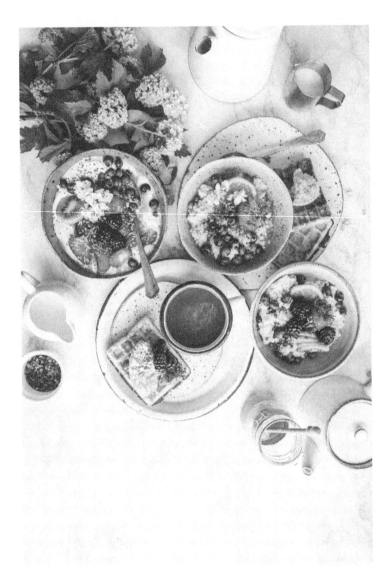

# Egg White and Broccoli Omelette

## DESCRIPTION:

A light, tasty and incredibly fluffy omelette with egg whites, broccoli and a bit of extra cheese on top that is perfect for brunch or breakfast. Ready in just 5 minutes.

## INGREDIENTS FOR 2 SERVINGS

- 4 egg whites

- 1/3 cup of boiled broccoli

- ½ tsp of Dill

- 1 tbsp of parmesan cheese, grated

- Salt/Pepper

## METHOD

1. In a small bowl, beat together the egg whites until stiff and white.

2. Add the dill, the broccoli, and the parmesan cheese and incorporate everything with a spatula (do not over whisk).

3. Spray the pan with a bit of cooking spray and pour the egg and broccoli mixture. Cook around 1-2 minutes on each side.

4. Turn the omelette in half and optionally garnish with just a little bit of cheese on top.

**NUTRITIONAL INFORMATION (Per Serving)**

- Calories: 56.82 kcal
- Carbohydrate: 2.7 g
- Protein: 10.57 g
- Sodium: 271.9 mg
- Potassium: 168.74 mg
- Phosphorus: 50.8 mg
- Dietary Fiber: 0.79 g
- Fat: 1.65 g

# Yogurt Parfait with Strawberries

## DESCRIPTION

Do you need something fresh and sweet for breakfast? If yes, you can try this yogurt parfait with strawberries that will be ready in a minute and it is loaded with vanilla powder for extra protein.

## INGREDIENTS FOR 2 SERVINGS

- ½ cup of soy yogurt (plain)
- 1 scoop of vanilla flavored protein
- 5 fresh strawberries, sliced
- 1 tbsp of agave syrup

## METHOD

1. In a bowl, slowly whisk the protein powder with the yogurt.

2. Add the strawberry slices and the agave syrup on top.

3. Serve.

## NUTRITIONAL INFORMATION (Per Serving)

- Calories: 153.25 kcal
- Carbohydrate: 23.5 g
- Protein: 12.67 g
- Sodium: 93.32 mg
- Potassium: 85.9 mg
- Phosphorus: 62.75 mg
- Dietary Fiber: 1.43 g
- Fat: 1.17 g

# Mexican Scrambled eggs in tortilla

## DESCRIPTION

A hearty egg recipe inspired by the true Mexican flavors of chillies and cumin, which is easy to make and has an incredible taste. Perfect for a brunch for two.

## INGREDIENTS FOR 2 SERVINGS

- 2 medium corn tortillas

- 4 egg whites

- 1 tsp of cumin

- 3 tsp of green chillies, diced

- ½ tsp of hot pepper sauce

- 2 tbsp of salsa

- ½ tsp salt

## METHOD

1. Spray some cooking spray on a medium skillet and heat for a few seconds.
2. Whisk the eggs with the green chillies, hot sauce and cumin.
3. Add the eggs into the pan, and whisk with a spatula to scrumble. Add the salt.
4. Cook until fluffy and done (1-2 minutes) over low heat.
5. Open the tortillas and spread 1 tbsp of salsa on each.
6. Distribute the egg mixture onto the tortillas and wrap gently to make a burrito.
7. Serve warm.

## NUTRITIONAL INFORMATION (Per Serving)

- Calories: 44.1 kcal
- Carbohydrate: 2.23 g
- Protein: 7.69 g
- Sodium: 854 mg
- Potassium: 189 mg

- Phosphorus: 22 mg
- Dietary Fiber: 0.5 g
- Fat: 0.39 g

# American Blueberry Pancakes

## DESCRIPTION

Everyone loves good old-pancakes that reminds us of those that our grandmas used to make. The addition of blueberries here adds a nice tangy twist while keeping phosphorus and potassium levels low.

## INGREDIENTS FOR 6 SERVINGS

- 1 ½ cups of all-purpose flour, sifted

- 1 cup of buttermilk

- 3 tbsp of sugar

- 2 tbsp of unsalted butter, melted

- 2 tsp of baking powder

- 2 eggs, beaten

- 1 cup of canned blueberries, rinsed

## METHOD

1. Combine the flour, baking powder and sugar in a bowl.
2. Make a hole in the center and slowly add the rest of the ingredients.
3. Begin to stir gently from the sides to the center with a spatula, until you get a smooth and creamy batter.
4. Spray a small pan with cooking spray and place over medium heat.
5. Take one measuring cup and fill 1/3rd of its capacity with the batter to make each pancake.
6. Use a spoon to pour the pancake batter and let cook until golden brown. Flip once to cook the other side.
7. Serve warm with optional agave syrup.

## NUTRITIONAL INFORMATION (Per Serving)

- Calories: 251.69 kcal
- Carbohydrate: 41.68 g
- Protein: 7.2 g

- Sodium: 186.68 mg
- Potassium: 142.87 mg
- Phosphorus: 255.39 mg
- Dietary Fiber: 1.9 g
- Fat: 6.47 g

# Raspberry Peach Breakfast Smoothie

## COOKING TIME: 1 MINUTE

**DESCRIPTION**

A bright, rich, and zesty smoothie for kick-starting your day with energy and nutrients that will keep you until lunch.

**INGREDIENTS FOR 2 SERVINGS**

- 1/3 cup of raspberries, (it can be frozen)

- 1/2 peach, skin and pit removed

- 1 tbsp of honey

- 1 cup of coconut water

**METHOD**

1. Combine all the ingredients together in a blender until smooth.
2. Pour and serve chilled in a tall glass or mason jar.

## NUTRITIONAL INFORMATION (Per Serving)

- Calories: 86.3 kcal
- Carbohydrate: 20.6 g
- Protein: 1.4 g
- Sodium: 3 mg
- Potassium: 109 mg
- Phosphorus: 36.08 mg
- Dietary Fiber: 2.6 g
- Fat: 0.31 g

# Fast Microwave Egg Scramble

## DESCRIPTION

Do you need your eggs extra fast without getting stuff dirty? You can try this 1 ½ minute scramble microwave recipe that is low in phosphorus and moderate to low in potassium levels as well.

## INGREDIENTS FOR 1 SERVING

- 1 large egg

- 2 large egg whites

- 2 tbsp of milk

- Kosher pepper, ground

## DIRECTIONS

1. Spray a coffee cup with a bit of cooking spray.

2. Whisk all the ingredients together and place into the coffee cup.
3. Place the cup with the eggs into the microwave and set to cook for approx. 45 seconds. Take out and stir.
4. Return to the microwave and cook for another 30 seconds.
5. Serve.

**NUTRITIONAL INFORMATION (Per Serving)**

- Calories: 128.6 kcal
- Carbohydrate: 2.47 g
- Protein: 12.96 g
- Sodium: 286.36 mg
- Potassium: 185.28 mg
- Phosphorus: 122.22 mg
- Dietary Fiber: 0 g
- Fat: 5.96 g

# Mango Lassi Smoothie

## DESCRIPTION

This smoothie recipe stands out from the rest in its rich exotic aroma and zesty flavor, thanks to a smart combination of mango and spices like cinnamon and cardamom. Great for breakfast or post or pre-workout snack.

## INGREDIENTS FOR 1-2 SERVINGS

- ½ cup of plain yogurt

- ½ cup of plain water

- ½ cup of sliced mango

- 1 tbsp of sugar

- ¼ tsp of cardamom

- ¼ tsp cinnamon

- ¼ cup lime juice

## METHOD

1. Pulse all the above ingredients in a blender until smooth (around 1 minute).
2. Pour into tall glasses or mason jars and serve chilled immediately.

## NUTRITIONAL INFORMATION (Per Serving)

- Calories: 89.02 kcal
- Carbohydrate: 14.31 g
- Protein: 2.54 g
- Sodium: 30 mg
- Potassium: 185.67 mg
- Phosphorus: 67.88 mg
- Dietary Fiber: 0.77 g
- Fat: 2.05 g

# Breakfast Maple Sausage

## DESCRIPTION

If you are a meat lover, you will simply love this rich breakfast sausage recipe that is high in protein but low in phosphorus and potassium. You can also keep any leftovers of this for casseroles, omelettes, and sandwiches.

## INGREDIENTS FOR 12 SERVINGS

- 1 pound of pork, minced

- ½ pound lean turkey meat, ground

- ¼ tsp of nutmeg

- ½ tsp black pepper

- ¼ all spice

- 2 tbsp of maple syrup

- 1 tbsp of water

## METHOD

1. Combine all the ingredients in a bowl.

2. Cover and place in the fridge for 3-4 hours.

3. Take the mixture and form into small flat patties with your hand (around 10-12 patties).

4. Lightly grease a medium skillet with oil and shallow fry the patties over medium to high heat, until brown (around 4-5 minutes on each side).

5. Serve hot.

## NUTRITIONAL INFORMATION (Per Serving)

- Calories: 53.85 kcal
- Carbohydrate: 2.42 g
- Protein: 8.5 g
- Sodium: 30.96 mg
- Potassium: 84.68 mg
- Phosphorus: 83.49 mg
- Dietary Fiber: 0.03 g
- Fat: 0.9 g

# Summer Veggie Omelette

## DESCRIPTION

This blend of summer veggies like zucchini, corn, and fresh onions helps you to realize how rich and nutrient dense can omelette be. It's so filling that you won't need anything else other than a smoothie or tea for breakfast.

## INGREDIENTS FOR 1-2 SERVINGS

- 4 large egg whites

- ¼ cup of sweet corn, frozen

- ⅓ cup of zucchini, grated

- 2 green onions, sliced

- 1 tbsp of cream cheese

- Kosher pepper

## METHOD

1. Grease a medium pan with some cooking spray and add the onions, corn and grated zucchini.
2. Saute for a couple of minutes until softened.
3. Beat the eggs together with the water, cream cheese, and pepper in a bowl.
4. Add the eggs into the veggie mixture in the pan, and let cook while moving the edges from inside to outside with a spatula, to allow raw egg to cook through the edges.
5. Flip the omelette with the help of a dish (placed over the pan and flipped upside down and then back to the pan).
6. Let sit for another 1-2 minutes.
7. Fold in half and serve.

## NUTRITIONAL INFORMATION (Per Serving)

- Calories: 90 kcal
- Carbohydrate: 15.97 g
- Protein: 8.07 g

- Sodium: 227 mg
- Potassium: 244..24 mg
- Phosphorus: 45.32 mg
- Dietary Fiber: 0.88 g
- Fat: 2.44 g

# Raspberry Overnight Porridge

## DESCRIPTION

Many people dislike the texture of warm porridge alone but there is a delicious version of the good old porridge. In this recipe, the oats are soaked in the almond milk overnight so they get soft and ready to enjoy the next morning.

## INGREDIENTS FOR 1 SERVING

- ⅓ cup of rolled oats

- ½ cup almond milk

- 1 tbsp of honey

- 5-6 raspberries, fresh or canned and unsweetened

## METHOD

1. Combine the oats, almond milk, and honey in a mason jar and place into the fridge for overnight.
2. Serve the next morning with the raspberries on top.

**NUTRITIONAL INFORMATION (Per Serving)**

- Calories: 143.6 kcal
- Carbohydrate: 34.62 g
- Protein: 3.44 g
- Sodium: 77.88 mg
- Potassium: 153.25 mg
- Phosphorus: 99.3 mg
- Dietary Fiber: 7.56 g
- Fat: 3.91 g

# Lunch

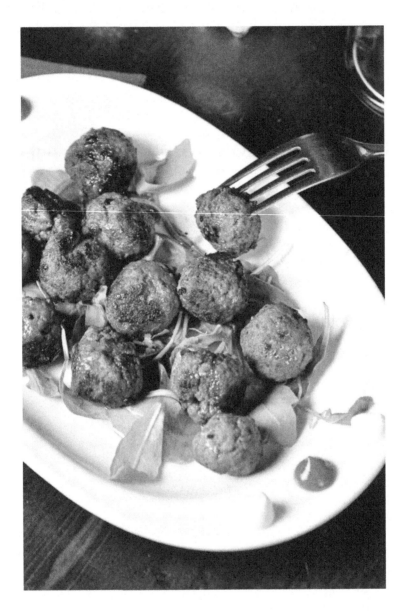

# Light Beef Enchiladas

## DESCRIPTION

Enchiladas are a classic Mexican favorite for many; however, they can be hidden calorie and fat bombs. This recipe is much leaner yet equally delicious and, it has moderate to low amounts of potassium.

## INGREDIENTS FOR 6 SERVING

### (12 enchiladas).

- 1 pound (around 650 grams) ground lean beef

- ½ cup shallots, chopped

- 1 clove of garlic

- 1 tsp of ground cumin

- ½ tsp cayenne pepper

- 1 can or small (200-gram jar) of enchilada sauce

- 12 corn tortillas

- A bit of low extra cheese on top (optional)

- Kosher pepper

## METHOD

1. In a medium frying pan with 1 tsp of oil, brown the ground beef and the shallots (around 5-6 minutes).

2. Add the garlic and spices and toss to mix well. Cook until meat will become brown and shallots will be soft and transparent. Add half of the enchilada sauce toss and cook for another 5 minutes.

3. Lightly toast the corn tortillas for 30-40 seconds on the toaster.

4. Distribute in each the remaining enchilada sauce and the ground beef

mixture. Wrap and roll from one side to another to make enchiladas.

5. Sprinkle optionally a bit of grated cheddar cheese on top and place in the microwave for 1-2 minutes to melt the cheese and serve.

## NUTRITIONAL INFORMATION (Per Serving)

- Calories: 286.70 kcal
- Carbohydrate: 30.75 g
- Protein: 26.3 g
- Sodium: 201.91 mg
- Potassium: 224.35 mg
- Phosphorus: 146.39 mg
- Dietary Fiber: 3.8 g
- Fat: 9 g

# Creamy Chicken with Cider

## DESCRIPTION

An easy 4-ingredient recipe that is full of flavor and is ready in under 30 minutes. Great as a family lunch on weekends or even as a hearty guest dish. It has a light gravy sauce for that extra dose of flavor.

## INGREDIENTS FOR 8 SERVINGS

- 4 bone-in chicken breasts

- 2 tbsp of lightly salted butter

- ¾ cup apple cider vinegar

- ⅔ cup of rich unsweetened coconut milk or cream

- Kosher pepper

## METHOD

1. Melt the butter in a skillet over medium heat.

2. Season the chicken with the pepper and add to the skillet. Cook over low heat for approx. 20 minutes.
3. Remove the chicken from the heat and set aside in a dish.
4. In the same skillet, add the cider and bring to a boil until most of it has evaporated.
5. Add the coconut cream and let cook for 1 minute until slightly thickened.
6. Pour the cider cream over the cooked chicken and serve.

## NUTRITIONAL INFORMATION (Per Serving)

- Calories: 86.76 kcal
- Carbohydrate: 1.88 g
- Protein: 1.5 g
- Sodium: 93.52 mg
- Potassium: 74.65 mg
- Phosphorus: 36.54 mg
- Dietary Fiber: 0.1 g
- Fat: 8.21 g

# Easy and Fast Mac-n-Cheese

## COOKING TIME: 8-10 MINUTES

### DESCRIPTION

Mac-n-cheese is favorite soul food for kids and adults alike. It's not what we call "healthy" as it is loaded with a high amount of carbs but when on a renal diet, this is fine as it is very low in potassium and phosphorus.

### INGREDIENTS FOR 4 SERVINGS

- 1 cup of dry elbow macaroni pasta

- ½ cup of mild cheddar cheese

- 3 cups of water

- 1 tsp of unsalted butter

- ½ tsp of dry mustard powder

- ½ tsp of paprika

### METHOD

1. Boil the elbow macaroni in boiling water for 7-8 minutes (or until soft).
2. Drain all the water out and transfer in the bowl.
3. Add the butter cheese, mustard, and paprika while the pasta is still hot, toss and serve.

**NUTRITIONAL INFORMATION (Per Serving)**

- Calories: 231.68 kcal
- Carbohydrate: 32.65 g
- Protein: 9.74 g
- Sodium: 107.25 mg
- Potassium: 29.52 mg
- Phosphorus: 159.93 mg
- Dietary Fiber: 0.12 g
- Fat: 7.2 g

# *Italian Meatballs*

## DESCRIPTION

Italian meatballs are renowned for their mild aromatic flavor and solid texture that blends ideally with a light tomato sauce. If you wish to try a low sodium alternative to this classic Italian dish, try this recipe.

## INGREDIENTS FOR 12 SERVINGS

- 1.5 pounds of ground beef chuck,

- 2 eggs, beaten

- ½ cup of red onion, chopped

- ½ cup of rolled oat flakes

- ½ tsp of garlic salt

- 1 tsp of dried oregano

- 3 tbsp of parmesan cheese

- 1 tbsp of tomato paste

- ½ tsp of black pepper

**METHOD**

1. Preheat your oven at 375 F/190C.
2. Mix all the ingredients in a large bowl.
3. Shape into small balls (around 1 inch) and place on a Pyrex or baking sheet.
4. Bake for 15-17 minutes (or until they are fully cooked and slightly brown on the outside).
5. Remove from the oven and serve with a light tomato sauce or hot sauce and rice.

**NUTRITIONAL INFORMATION (Per Serving)**

- Calories: 133.12 kcal
- Carbohydrate: 5.8 g
- Protein: 14.4 g
- Sodium: 62.76 mg
- Potassium: 252.67 mg
- Phosphorus: 166.65 mg
- Dietary Fiber: 0.89 g
- Fat: 5.3 g

# Exotic Palabok

## DESCRIPTION

A delicious recipe from the Philippines that combines the flavors of rice noodles and shrimp.

## INGREDIENTS FOR 6 SERVINGS

- 12 oz. rice noodles.

- 1 ½ cups of medium shrimp, peeled and deveined

- ⅔ cup white onion, chopped

- 1 spring onion, sliced

- 3 tbsp of canola oil

- 1 pound, lean ground turkey

- 2 cups firm tofu, chopped

- 2 packs of shrimp or ordinary gravy mix

- 5 hard boiled eggs

- 1 lemon

- ½ cup of pork rinds (optional)

## METHOD

1. Boil rice noodles until nice and soft. Keep aside.
2. Boil the peeled shrimp for 2-3 minutes in a pot with plain water.
3. In a wok or shallow pan, saute the garlic and onion with the oil. Add the ground turkey, tofu and shrimps.
4. Dissolve the gravy mix in water or as per package instructions.
5. Combine the rice noodles, tofu, onions and the gravy mix with ½ cup of pork rind (optional).
6. Slice the egg and lemons.
7. Serve with egg and lemons on top.

## NUTRITIONAL INFORMATION (Per Serving)

- Calories: 305 kcal
- Carbohydrate: 39.14 g
- Protein: 17.6 g
- Sodium: 536 mg
- Potassium: 243.52 mg
- Phosphorus: 180.41 mg
- Dietary Fiber: 0.9 g
- Fat: 9 g

# Vegetarian Gobi Curry

## DESCRIPTION

An ethnic Indian recipe that comes from the Gobi desert area with a creamy and spicy flavor and texture that is a comfort for everyone. Vegetarians will love this recipe, as it's quite delicious and filling.

## INGREDIENTS

- 2 cups of cauliflower florets

- 2 tbsp of unsalted butter

- 1 medium dry white onion, thinly chopped

- ½ cup of green peas(frozen if wish)

- 1 tsp of fresh ginger, chopped

- 1/2 tsp of turmeric

- 1 tsp of garam masala

- ¼ tsp cayenne pepper

- 1 tbsp of water

**METHOD**

1. Heat a skillet over medium heat with the butter and saute the onions until caramelized (golden brown).
2. Add the spices e.g. ginger, garam masala turmeric and cayenne.
3. Add the cauliflower and the (frozen) peas and stir.
4. Add the water and cover with a lid. Reduce the heat to a low temperature and let cook covered for 10 minutes.
5. Serve with white rice.

**NUTRITIONAL INFORMATION (Per Serving)**

- Calories: 91.04 kcal
- Carbohydrate: 7.3 g
- Protein: 2.19 g
- Sodium: 39.38 mg
- Potassium: 209.58 mg

- Phosphorus: 42 mg
- Dietary Fiber: 3 g
- Fat: 6.4 g

# Marinated Shrimp and Pasta

COOKING TIME: 10 MINUTES

## DESCRIPTION

A hearty recipe that combines shrimps, pasta and various veggies for a burst of colors and flavors. A great pasta salad dish for lunch and guest food.

## INGREDIENTS FOR 10 SERVINGS

- 12 oz. of three-colored penne pasta

- ½ pound of cooked shrimp

- ½ red bell pepper, diced

- ½ cup of red onion, chopped

- 3 stalks of celery

- 12 baby carrots, cut into thick slices

- 1 cup of cauliflower, cut into small round pieces

- ¼ cup of honey

- ¼ cup balsamic vinegar

- ½ tsp of black pepper

- ½ tsp garlic powder

- 1 tbsp of French mustard

- ¾ cup of olive oil

## METHOD

1. Cook pasta for around 10 minutes (or according to packaged instructions).

2. While pasta is boiling, cut all your veggies and place into a large mixing bowl. Add the cooked shrimp.

3. In a mixing bowl, add the honey, vinegar, black pepper, garlic powder, and mustard.

4. While you whisk, slowly incorporate the oil and stir well.

5. Add in the drained pasta with the veggies and shrimp and gently combine everything together.
6. Pour the liquid marinade over the pasta and veggies and toss to coat everything evenly.
7. Refrigerate for 3-5 hours prior to serving.
8. Serve chilled.

**NUTRITIONAL INFORMATION (Per Serving)**

- Calories: 256 kcal
- Carbohydrate: 41 g
- Protein: 6.55 g
- Sodium:242.04 mg
- Potassium: 131.88 mg
- Phosphorus: 86.03 mg
- Dietary Fiber: 2.28 g
- Fat: 16.88 g

# *Steak and Onion Sandwich*

## DESCRIPTION

A rich steak sandwich that is very filling when you have to eat something good but don't have much time. Make this ahead for next working day lunch or enjoy it fresh with the rest of your family.

## INGREDIENTS FOR 4 SERVINGS

- 4 flank steaks (around 4 oz. each)

- 1 medium red onion, sliced

- 1 tbsp of lemon juice

- 1 tbsp of Italian seasoning

- 1 tsp of black pepper

- 1 tbsp of vegetable oil

- 4 sandwich/burger buns

## METHOD

1. Wrap the steak with the lemon juice, the Italian seasoning, and pepper to taste. Cut into 4 pieces
2. Heat the vegetable oil in a medium skillet over medium heat.
3. Cook steaks around 3 minutes on each side until you get a medium to well-done result. Take off and transfer onto a dish with absorbing paper.
4. In the same skillet, saute the onions until tender and transparent (around 3 minutes).
5. Cut the sandwich bun into half and place 1 piece of steak in each topped with the onions.
6. Serve or wrap with paper or foil and keep in the fridge for the next day.

## NUTRITIONAL INFORMATION (Per Serving)

- Calories: 315.26 kcal
- Carbohydrate: 8.47 g

- Protein: 38.33 g
- Sodium: 266.24 mg
- Potassium: 238.2 mg
- Phosphorus: 364.25 mg
- Dietary Fiber: 0.76 g
- Fat: 13.22 g

# *Zesty Crab Cakes*

## DESCRIPTION

Crab cakes are a favorite dish in American seafood restaurants and are loved by kids and adults alike. If you like crab cakes, try this tasty recipe guilty-free as it is quite low on phosphorus and potassium.

## INGREDIENTS FOR 6 SERVINGS

- 9 oz. (250 grams) of crab meat

- ⅓ cup green or red bell pepper, thinly chopped

- ⅓ cup low salt crackers, crushed

- ¼ cup low-fat mayonnaise

- 1 tbsp of dry mustard

- ½ tsp of pepper

- 2 tbsp of lemon juice

- ½ tsp of lemon zest

- 1 tsp of garlic powder

- 2 tbsp of vegetable oil

**METHOD**

1. Mix all the ingredients except for the oil until uniform. Divide into 6 flat patties (around 5 inches in diameter).
2. Heat the vegetable oil in the skillet and shallow fry the patties for 2-3 minutes on each side (or until golden brown).
3. Serve warm on a dish with absorbing paper.

**NUTRITIONAL INFORMATION (Per Serving)**

- Calories: 144.42 kcal
- Carbohydrate: 5.12 g
- Protein: 8.47 g
- Sodium: 212.31 mg
- Potassium: 195 mg
- Phosphorus: 127.42 mg

- Dietary Fiber: 1.02 g
- Fat: 9.2 g

# Stuffed Green Peppers

## DESCRIPTION

Green peppers are very delicious stuffed with rice and ground meat. This recipe calls for ground chicken or turkey and rice for a delicious yet light combo that is low in fat, potassium, and phosphorus.

## INGREDIENTS FOR 6 SERVINGS

- 6 small to medium green peppers, seeds, and tops removed

- ½ pound of lean turkey or sausage meat

- ¼ cup red onions, chopped

- ¼ cup celery stalks, chopped

- 1 ½ cup of cooked white rice

- 2 tbsp of lemon juice

- 2 tbsp of Italian seasoning

- ½ tsp of black pepper

- ½ tsp of sugar

- 2 tbsp of vegetable oil

## METHOD

1. Preheat the oven at 325F /180C.
2. Heat the vegetable oil in the pan.
3. Add in the pan the ground chicken, celery, onions, and cook until meat is become lightly brown (around 6-7 minutes).
4. Add all the remaining ingredients except peppers to the pan. Stir everything together and take off the heat.
5. Transfer and divide the mixture into the open green peppers. Place in a baking dish, cover and bake for 30 minutes.
6. Serve hot.

## NUTRITIONAL INFORMATION (Per Serving)

- Calories: 137.8 kcal

- Carbohydrate: 18.5 g
- Protein: 5.2 g
- Sodium: 182.65 mg
- Potassium: 251.36 mg
- Phosphorus: 64.97 mg
- Dietary Fiber: 3.5 g
- Fat: 5.2 g

# Dinner

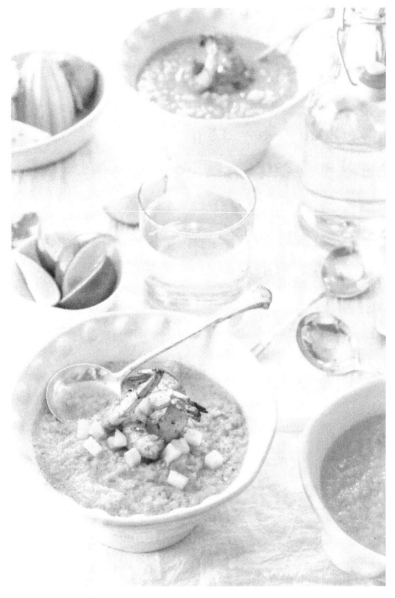

# *Chicken and Noodle Soup*

## COOKING TIME: 45 MINUTES

## DESCRIPTION

A hearty recipe for the cold nights where you want something delicious and warm. The recipe is incredibly low in potassium and phosphorus so feel free to have a second bowl of this.

## INGREDIENTS FOR 8 SERVINGS

- 1 pound of cut chicken parts e.g. thighs, breast, wings, etc.

- ¼ cup of lemon juice

- 3 ½ cups of water

- ½ cup of green pepper, diced

- ½ cup of celery, sliced

- 1 cup of egg noodles

- 1 tbsp of chicken seasoning

- 1 tsp of garlic powder

- 1 tsp of onion powder

- 1 tsp of red cayenne pepper

- 1 tsp of sugar

- 2 tbsp of vegetable oil

**METHOD**

1. Rub the chicken pieces with the lemon juice.
2. Combine chicken, water, chicken seasoning and the rest of the spices with the sugar together.
3. Bring to a boil and let cook for 30 minutes or until chicken is fully cooked and tender.
4. Add the pepper and noodles and cook for an extra 15 minutes.
5. Serve hot.

**NUTRITIONAL INFORMATION (Per Serving)**

- Calories: 66.45 kcal
- Carbohydrate: 6.92 g
- Protein: 1.29 g
- Sodium: 6.97 mg
- Potassium: 52.08 mg
- Phosphorus: 26.26 mg
- Dietary Fiber: 0.68 g
- Fat: 3.99 g

# Barbeque Turkey Cups

## COOKING TIME: 12 MINUTES

**METHOD**

Try this delicious recipe of cups filled with turkey and barbeque sauce that is also very easy to make.

**INGREDIENTS FOR 10 SERVINGS**

- A 10 oz. package of frozen low-fat biscuits

- ¾ pounds of lean ground turkey breast

- ½ cup of mildly hot and spicy barbeque sauce

- 2 tsp of onion flakes

- ½ tsp of garlic powder

- 1 tbsp of vegetable oil

**METHOD**

1. Heat the oil in the skillet and add the ground turkey with the garlic powder, and cook until brown.
2. Add the onion flakes and the barbeque sauce and stir well.
3. Flatten each biscuit with a spatula and press into a muffin tin.
4. Distribute the barbeque/turkey mixture with a spoon to stuff each muffin.
5. Bake at 400 F/190 C in the oven for 10-12 minutes.

**NUTRITIONAL INFORMATION (Per Serving)**

- Calories: 178.15 kcal
- Carbohydrate: 16.92 g
- Protein: 11.28 g
- Sodium: 1660.32 mg
- Potassium: 178.3 mg
- Phosphorus: 203.57 mg
- Dietary Fiber: 0.71 g
- Fat: 7.15 g

# Low Sodium Green Bean Casserole

## DESCRIPTION

A holiday favorite dish made lighter with less sodium and fat yet still delicious and hearty with a bit of a light crunch. You may cook this for dinner and then keep any leftovers for the next day.

## INGREDIENTS FOR 8-10 SERVINGS

- 24 oz. of frozen green beans, thawed and cooked

- 1 red onion, chopped

- 2 garlic cloves, minced

- 1 cup of panko breadcrumbs

- ½ pound of fresh mushrooms, thinly sliced

- 3 cups of simple white/béchamel sauce (cooked with 4 tbsp of butter, 4 tbsp of flour and 4 cups of milk).

## METHOD

1. Preheat your oven at 350F/180.
2. Melt in a skillet the butter and mix with breadcrumbs. Keep aside.
3. Saute the garlic and the onions in the remaining amount of butter until transparent and softened.
4. Add the sliced mushrooms and cook until soft (around 8 minutes).
5. In a lightly greased baking dish combine the green beans with the mushrooms and the cooked white sauce and stir well.
6. Top with the breadcrumbs and bake for 20-25 minutes or until golden brown on top.

## NUTRITIONAL INFORMATION (Per Serving)

- Calories: 161.74 kcal

- Carbohydrate: 21.3 g
- Protein: 6.22 g
- Sodium: 322.53 mg
- Potassium: 233.37 mg
- Phosphorus: 140.3 mg
- Dietary Fiber:  5.53 g
- Fat: 6.94 g

# Marinated Mushrooms in the Broiler

## DESCRIPTION

Portobello mushrooms have a rich flavor and texture that almost resembles meat-especially if you cook them on the grill. You may try this broiler version that will be delicious.

## INGREDIENTS FOR 5-6 SERVINGS

- 3 large Portobello mushrooms

- 1/3 cup of shallots, finely chopped

- 3 tbsp of balsamic vinegar

- ⅓ of brown sugar

- 3 tbsp of sesame oil

- 2 tbsp of low sodium soy sauce

## METHOD

1. Wash the mushrooms, rinse and set aside.

2. Combine all the rest ingredients in a bowl to make a marinade. Add the mushrooms and let marinate in the fridge for at least 3 hours or overnight.

3. Place the mushrooms on a baking dish and cook in the broiler for 12-15 minutes.

4. Let the mushrooms rest for two minutes prior to serving.

## NUTRITIONAL INFORMATION (Per Serving)

- Calories: 106.27 kcal
- Carbohydrate: 6.82 g
- Protein: 2.03 g
- Sodium: 212.98 mg
- Potassium: 196.75 mg
- Phosphorus: 74.8 mg
- Dietary Fiber: 1.18 g
- Fat: 8.58 g

# *Italian Style Lamb Patties*

## DESCRIPTION

A nice aromatic patty dish inspired by the flavors and aromas of the Italian and Mediterranean cuisine; oregano, feta, and garlic blend nicely with the lamb without overpowering its original taste.

## INGREDIENTS FOR 12 SERVINGS

- 1 lb of ground lean lamb

- ½ cup of feta cheese, crumbled

- 1 clove of garlic, minced

- ½ tsp of dried oregano

- ½ tsp of crushed black pepper

- ¼ cup of white onion, chopped

- ¼ cup of panko breadcrumbs

## METHOD

1. Combine the lamb with all the ingredients in a large bowl.
2. Shape into 4 patties of equal size (around ½ inch thick).
3. Heat a grilling and non-stick pan over medium heat with cooking spray.
4. Add the lamb patties and let them cook on high heat for nearly 5 minutes on each side. Ensure that the patties are no pink in the center by cutting one in half.
5. Serve

## NUTRITIONAL INFORMATION (Per Serving)

- Calories: 118.39 kcal
- Carbohydrate: 2.1 g
- Protein: 7.5 g
- Sodium: 88.4 mg
- Potassium: 9.93 mg
- Phosphorus: 21.82 mg
- Dietary Fiber: 0.8 g
- Fat: 9.2 g

# Chicken with Jalapeno

## DESCRIPTION

An easy chicken recipe spiced up with the flavors of jalapeno pepper, nutmeg, and black pepper. The added chicken stock makes this extra juicy and flavorsome.

## INGREDIENTS FOR 8 SERVINGS

- 2 ½ pounds of chicken pieces, skin and fat removed

- 1 onion, cut into rings

- 1 ½ cups of chicken stock

- 1/2 tsp of ground nutmeg

- 2 tsp of jalapeno peppers, chopped and seeds removed

- 2 tbsp of vegetable oil

## METHOD

1. Heat the oil in the skillet and add the chicken pieces. Cook until brown and set aside.

2. Add the onion rings to the skillet with the oil and add the chicken stock, stirring occasionally.

3. Place the chicken pieces back to the pan. Add the pepper and nutmeg.

4. Cover the pan and let cook on low heat for 25-30 minutes.

5. Add the jalapeno peppers and cook for another two minutes.

6. Serve.

**NUTRITIONAL INFORMATION (Per Serving)**

- Calories: 256.18 kcal
- Carbohydrate: 1.79 g
- Protein: 31.1 g
- Sodium: 176.5 mg
- Potassium: 169.74 mg
- Phosphorus: 309.55 mg
- Dietary Fiber: 0.9 g
- Fat: 13.15 g

# Easy Mexican Soup

## DESCRIPTION

If you love Mexican flavors but don't want to go for something solid to ease your hunger, you may try this soup with corn and black beans that are so easy to make.

## INGREDIENTS FOR 6 SERVINGS

- 1/3 cup of black beans (low fat)

- 1 can of sweet corn

- 1 tbsp of tomato paste

- 1 can of chicken bouillon soup

- 4 cups of water

- 2 boneless chicken thighs, skin and fat removed, chopped

## METHOD

1. Mix all the ingredients together in a pot and let cook on low heat for 30-35 minutes.
2. Serve hot.

**NUTRITIONAL INFORMATION (Per Serving)**

- Calories: 221.5 kcal
- Carbohydrate: 11.9 g
- Protein: 15 g
- Sodium: 323.98 mg
- Potassium: 337.65 mg
- Phosphorus: 170.8 mg
- Dietary Fiber: 2.26 g
- Fat: 13 g

# *Seafood Casserole*

## DESCRIPTION

A delicious casserole recipe made with crabmeat, tuna, and shrimps blended nicely with veggies for that extra flavor and crunch. Very low in fat, sodium, and phosphorus.

## INGREDIENTS FOR 6 SERVINGS

- 1 cup of crab meat, boiled

- 1 cup of medium to small shrimp, boiled

- 4 tbsp of green pepper, diced

- ½ cup of frozen green peas

- 2 tbsp of green onions, chopped

- 1 cup of celery, sliced

- ½ cup of low-fat mayonnaise

- 1 cup of regular breadcrumbs

**METHOD**

1. Preheat the oven at 375F/180C.
2. Mix all the ingredients except for breadcrumbs in a mixing bowl. Stir and press lightly with a fork to make everything even.
3. Transfer the mixture into a greased casserole dish.
4. Place the breadcrumbs on top.
5. Bake for 25-20 minutes.

**NUTRITIONAL INFORMATION (Per Serving)**

- Calories: 225.1 kcal
- Carbohydrate: 18.17 g
- Protein: 16.4 g
- Sodium: 609.55 mg
- Potassium: 213.49 mg
- Phosphorus: 211.39 mg
- Dietary Fiber: 2.6 g
- Fat: 9.4 g

# Beef and Veggie Soup

## COOKING TIME: 50 MINUTES

**DESCRIPTION**

This soup recipe will remind you of the classic Sunday beef stew, as the ingredients are nearly the same but on a soup version. A lovely soup for the entire family.

**INGREDIENTS FOR 8 SERVING**

- 1 pound of beef pieces, for stew

- 2/3 cup of white onion, sliced

- ½ cup of frozen green peas

- ⅓ cup carrot, diced

- ½ of frozen corn kernels

- 3 ½ cups of water

- ½ tsp of dried basil

- ½ tsp of thyme

- 2 tbsp of olive oil

## METHOD

1. Grease the bottom of a large pot with olive oil and place the onions with all the fresh veggies, and saute for 3-4 minutes.
2. Add the frozen veggies, the meat and let simmer on low heat for 45-50 minutes.
3. Serve hot.

## NUTRITIONAL INFORMATION (Per Serving)

- Calories: 108.3 kcal
- Carbohydrate: 9.36 g
- Protein: 3.24 g
- Sodium: 233.57 mg
- Potassium: 167.97 mg
- Phosphorus: 43.42 mg
- Dietary Fiber: 1.4 g
- Fat: 6.7 g

# Pepper Linguini Pasta

## DESCRIPTION

Simple yet delicious recipe made with thin linguini pasta and roasted bell peppers for a bit of kick. The thyme and the butter add an extra dimension of flavor to this dish.

## INGREDIENTS FOR 7-8 SERVINGS

- 1 pack (16 0.z) of uncooked linguine pasta.

- ¾ cup of lightly salted butter

- 2 tbsp of fresh thyme

- 5 roasted red bell peppers, roughly chopped

- 3 cloves of garlic, minced

- 2 tbsp of olive oil

## METHOD

1. Fill half of a large pot with water and add the linguini pasta and olive oil. Allow cooking for 8-10 minutes (until softened). Drain and keep aside.

2. Heat two tbsp of butter in a pan over medium heat. Add the minced garlic and cook until golden brown. Add the rest of the butter, thyme and roasted bell peppers. Let cook until everything is heated evenly (around 2-3 minutes).

3. Serve the pepper sauce over the boiled pasta.

**NUTRITIONAL INFORMATION (Per Serving)**

- Calories: 407.75 kcal
- Carbohydrate: 50.11 g
- Protein: 8.78 g
- Sodium: 143.5 mg
- Potassium: 100.98 mg
- Phosphorus: 221.25 mg
- Dietary Fiber: 6.85 g
- Fat: 22.6 g

# *Desserts*

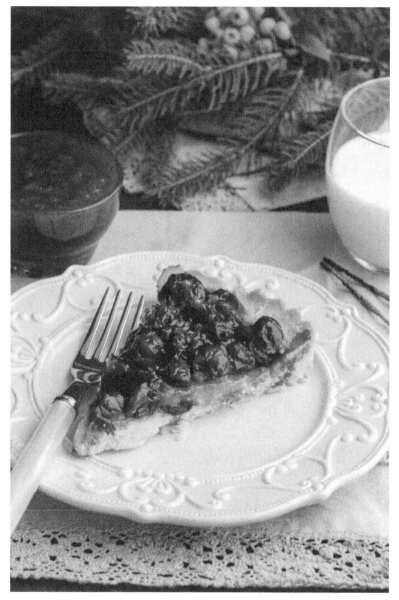

# Dessert Cocktail

## DESCRIPTION

A rich dessert and non-alcoholic cocktail made of forest fruits like cranberries and strawberries and sweetened with sugar, despite its rich flavor; it has 100 calories and is very low in potassium and phosphorus.

## INGREDIENTS FOR 4 SERVINGS

- 1 cup of cranberry juice

- 1 cup of fresh ripe strawberries, washed and hull removed

- 2 tbsp of lime juice

- ¼ cup of white sugar

- 8 ice cubes

## METHOD

1. Combine all the ingredients in a blender until smooth and creamy.
2. Pour the liquid into chilled tall glasses and serve cold.

## NUTRITIONAL INFORMATION (Per Serving)

- Calories: 92 kcal
- Carbohydrate: 23.5 g
- Protein: 0.5 g
- Sodium: 3.62 mg
- Potassium: 103.78 mg
- Phosphorus: 17.86 mg
- Dietary Fiber: 0.84 g
- Fat: 0.17 g

# Baked Egg Custard

## DESCRIPTION

A lovely and traditional egg custard recipe that you can enjoy on its own or as an extra in other dessert recipes. Very easy to make with just 5 ingredients.

## INGREDIENTS FOR 4 SERVINGS

- 2 medium eggs, at room temperature

- ¼ cup of semi-skimmed milk

- 3 tbsp of white sugar

- ½ tsp of nutmeg

- 1 tsp of vanilla extract

## METHOD

1. Preheat your oven at 375 F/180C

2. Mix all the ingredients in a mixing bowl and beat with a hand mixer for a few seconds until creamy and uniform.
3. Pour the mixture into lightly greased muffin tins.
4. Bake for 25-30 minutes or until the knife, you place inside, comes out clean.

**NUTRITIONAL INFORMATION (Per Serving)**

- Calories: 96.56 kcal
- Carbohydrate: 10.5 g
- Protein: 3.5 g
- Sodium: 37.75 mg
- Potassium: 58.19 mg
- Phosphorus: 58.76 mg
- Dietary Fiber: 0.06 g
- Fat: 2.91 g

# Gumdrop Cookies

## DESCRIPTION

A lively cookie recipe that is great for kids and will remind your childhood. If you have an upcoming kid's party, these cookies will be devoured in seconds.

## INGREDIENTS FOR 25 SERVINGS

## (50 cookies).

- ½ cup of spreadable unsalted butter

- 1 medium egg

- 1 cup of brown sugar

- 1 ⅔ cups of all-purpose flour, sifted

- ¼ cup of milk

- 1 tsp vanilla

- 1 tsp of baking powder

- 15 large gumdrops, chopped finely

**METHOD**

1. Preheat the oven at 400F/195C.
2. Combine the sugar, butter, and egg until creamy.
3. Add the milk and vanilla and stir well.
4. Combine the flour with the baking powder in a different bowl. Incorporate to the sugar, butter mixture, and stir.
5. Add the gumdrops and place the mixture in the fridge for half an hour.
6. Drop the dough with tablespoonful into a lightly greased baking or cookie sheet.
7. Bake for 10-12 minutes or until golden brown in color.

**NUTRITIONAL INFORMATION (Per Serving)**

- Calories: 102.17 kcal
- Carbohydrate: 16.5 g
- Protein: 0.86 g
- Sodium: 23.42 mg
- Potassium: 45 mg

- Phosphorus: 32.15 mg
- Dietary Fiber: 0.13 g
- Fat: 4 g

# *Pound Cake with Pineapple*

## DESCRIPTION

An old school cake recipe accentuated with the exotic flavors of pineapple for that sweet and slightly sour taste. Bake this and enjoy a same day or up to 5 days after baking.

## INGREDIENTS FOR 24 SERVINGS

## (1 cake/24 slice).

- 3 cups of all-purpose flour, sifted

- 3 cups of sugar

- 1 ½ cups of butter

- 6 whole eggs and 3 egg whites

- 1 tsp of vanilla extract

- 1 10.oz can of pineapple chunks, rinsed and crushed (keep juice aside).

**For the glaze:**

- 1 cup of sugar
- 1 stick of unsalted butter or margarine
- Reserved juice from the pineapple

## METHOD

1. Preheat the oven at 350F/180C.
2. Beat the sugar and the butter with a hand mixer until creamy and smooth.
3. Slowly add the eggs (one or two every time) and stir well after pouring each egg.
4. Add the vanilla extract, follow up with the flour and stir well.
5. Add the drained and chopped pineapple.
6. Pour the mixture into a greased cake tin and bake for 45-50 minutes.
7. In a small saucepan, combine the sugar with the butter and pineapple juice. Stir every few seconds and bring to boil. Cook until you get a creamy to thick glaze consistency.
8. Pour the glaze over the cake while still hot.

9. Let cook for at least 10 seconds and serve.

**NUTRITIONAL INFORMATION (Per Serving)**

- Calories: 407.4 kcal
- Carbohydrate: 79 g
- Protein: 4.25 g
- Sodium: 118.97 mg
- Potassium: 180.32 mg
- Phosphorus: 66.37 mg
- Dietary Fiber: 2.25 g
- Fat: 16.48 g

# Apple Crunch Pie

## DESCRIPTION

A lovely twist to the classic apple pie recipe with an added crunch on top of the apples. Made just with 6 ingredients and under 40 minutes. Feel free to serve this with a scoop of vanilla ice cream.

## INGREDIENTS FOR 8 SERVINGS

- 4 large tart apples, peeled, seeded and sliced

- ½ cup of white all-purpose flour

- ⅓ cup margarine

- 1 cup of sugar

- ¾ cup of rolled oat flakes

- ½ tsp of ground nutmeg

## METHOD

1. Preheat the oven to 375F/180C.

2. Place the apples over a lightly greased square pan (around 7 inches).

3. Mix the rest of the ingredients in a medium bowl with and spread the batter over the apples.

4. Bake for 30-35 minutes or until the top crust has gotten golden brown.

5. Serve hot.

## NUTRITIONAL INFORMATION (Per Serving)

- Calories: 261.9 kcal
- Carbohydrate: 47.2 g
- Protein: 1.5 g
- Sodium: 81 mg
- Potassium: 123.74 mg
- Phosphorus: 35.27 mg
- Dietary Fiber: 2.81 g
- Fat: 7.99 g

# Easy Chocolate Pie Shell

## DESCRIPTION

Do you wish to make an easy shell for your chocolate or custard pie from scratch? This recipe requires just 2 ingredients and it's so easy that even a kid can make.

## INGREDIENTS FOR 6 SERVINGS

**(6 servings/one empty pie crust).**

- 3 cups of cocoa rice Krispies, crushed
- ½ stick of unsalted butter, melted

## METHOD

1. Place crushed cocoa Krispies in a bowl with the melted butter. Mix well with a spatula.
2. Spray an 8-9 inch pie pan with some low-calorie cooking spray
3. Press the mixture into the pan and even out with a spatula.

4. Let sit and chill for at least 30 minutes in the fridge prior filling it with chocolate or vanilla pudding.

## NUTRITIONAL INFORMATION (Per Serving)

- Calories: 113.1 kcal
- Carbohydrate: 11.6 g
- Protein: 0.88 g
- Sodium: 122.98 mg
- Potassium: 17.3 mg
- Phosphorus: 18.23 mg
- Dietary Fiber: 0.04 g
- Fat: 7.82 g

# *Strawberry and Mint Sorbet*

## DESCRIPTION

Sorbets are probably one of the tangiest and refreshing desserts as they are fruity while containing low amounts of fat. Make this and enjoy alone or with other desserts.

## INGREDIENTS FOR 3-4 SERVINGS

- ¼ cup of white sugar

- 1 cup of frozen or fresh, sliced strawberries

- 1 tbsp of lime juice

- ¼ cup of water

- 1 ¼ cup of crushed ice

- A few mint leaves

## METHOD

1. Pulse and crush the ice in a heavy-duty blender.
2. Add the remaining ingredients and raise the speed to crush until no lumps of ice are left.
3. Optionally add a few mint leaves for garnishing.

## NUTRITIONAL INFORMATION (Per Serving)

- Calories: 93.34 kcal
- Carbohydrate: 32 g
- Protein: 0.33 g
- Sodium: 2.12 mg
- Potassium: 113.02 mg
- Phosphorus: 10.24 mg
- Dietary Fiber: 1.56 g
- Fat: 0.067 g

# Easy Chocolate Fudge

## DESCRIPTION

An old school fudge recipe will be easy to cook with just five ingredients and ready in 20 minutes (including cooling time). Make this ahead and keep for up two weeks at room temperature.

## INGREDIENTS FOR 12 SERVINGS

- ⅔ cup of half and half cream

- 1 cup of white granulated sugar

- 1 cups of semi-sweet chocolate chip cookies

- 1 cup of mini marshmallows

- 1 tsp of vanilla extract

## METHOD

1. Grease with cooking spray a square pie pan (around 9 inches).
2. Mix the half-and-half cream with the sugar in a medium saucepan. Bring to a boil and adjust to medium heat.
3. Take off the heat and add the chocolate chips, the marshmallows, and the vanilla extract. Stir well with a spatula until everything will be melted.
4. Quickly transfer the mixture into the pie pan. Let cool for at least 10 minutes and cut into square pieces, around 3x2" each. This will make 18-20 pieces.

**NUTRITIONAL INFORMATION (Per Serving)**

- Calories: 52.4 kcal
- Carbohydrate: 17.58 g
- Protein: 3.18 g
- Sodium: 153.47 mg
- Potassium: 100.52 mg
- Phosphorus: 38.63 mg
- Dietary Fiber: 1.35 g
- Fat: 21.3 g

# *High Protein Vanilla Cookies*

## DESCRIPTION

A delicious recipe with vanilla aromas amplified with extra whey protein powder and oatmeal for a bit of extra fiber. Enjoy and keep up to two weeks at room temperature.

## INGREDIENTS FOR 12 SERVINGS

## (24 cookies).

- ¾ cup of all-purpose flour

- ½ cup of oatmeal

- ½ cup of whey protein powder

- ¾ cups of brown sugar

- 1 egg

- 1 tsp of vanilla extract

- 1 tsp of baking soda

- 3 tbsp of margarine

**METHOD**

1. Preheat your oven at 325F/165C
2. Beat with the mixer the butter and the brown sugar.
3. Add the egg and the vanilla extract
4. Combine all the other ingredients until smooth (the mixture will be a tad drier than most cookie doughs).
5. Roll the batter with your hands into 1"balls.
6. Lightly grease a baking sheet and the cookie balls.
7. Bake for 10-12 minutes.

**NUTRITIONAL INFORMATION (Per Serving)**

- Calories: 292.95 kcal
- Carbohydrate: 29.1 g
- Protein: 35.1 g
- Sodium: 173.07 mg
- Potassium: 291.27 mg

- Phosphorus: 629.72 mg
- Dietary Fiber: 4.67 g
- Fat: 1.51 g

# Easy Pumpkin Pudding

## DESCRIPTION

If you love the festive flavors of pumpkin but don't want to get in the fuss of making a pumpkin pie, you can try this delicious and incredibly easy pumpkin pudding with just 5 ingredients.

## INGREDIENTS FOR 4 SERVINGS

- 3 oz. instant vanilla pudding mix powder

- 1 cup almond milk

- ½ cup of pumpkin puree

- 1 tsp of pumpkin spice mix

- 1 scoop of vanilla flavored protein powder

## METHOD

1. In a saucepan, mix the pudding mix and the almond milk.

2. Bring to a boil and reduce the heat as soon as the pudding has started to thicken.

3. Take off the heat and mix in the pumpkin puree, the pumpkin spice, and the protein powder. Stir well.

4. Transfer into a big glass bowl, let chill and cover with plastic wrap. Refrigerate for at least 5 hours prior to serving.

## NUTRITIONAL INFORMATION (Per Serving)

- Calories: 120.32 kcal
- Carbohydrate: 22.8 g
- Protein: 5.49 g
- Sodium: 370.66 mg
- Potassium: 84.44 mg
- Phosphorus: 164.57 mg
- Dietary Fiber: 0.9 g
- Fat: 0.84 g

# Conclusion

Renal diet may seem restricting for many, but in reality, there is plenty of low sodium, low phosphorus, and low potassium options to try out and we have proven it with this recipe book. Keep in mind that we have included roughly the levels of all these minerals in every recipe separately and therefore, you will have to calculate the total amounts you consume each day with all your daily meals.

Generally, most experts suggest up to 2700 mg of potassium and phosphorus per day for patients at the first two stages of renal disease while those at a more advanced stage should aim to consume up to 2000mg of these two minerals (each) per day to avoid dialysis. Since most of the recipes featured in this e-book contain up to 250 mg of potassium and phosphorus respectively, you can eat your breakfast, lunch, and dinner without worrying about crossing your daily limits.

Don't forget to do regular doctor check-ups to monitor your progress.

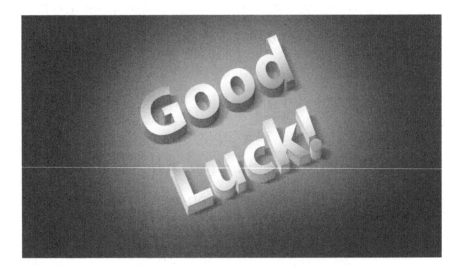

Made in the USA
Coppell, TX
29 October 2019